In 4 Weeks, Go Paleo

Paleolithic Dishes for Everyday Meals is a collection of Paleolithic dishes.

Shelia M. Britt

Contents

Chapter One

A Paleolithic Lifestyle in a Nutshell

Paleolithic is a term used to describe the period between the Stone Age and the present. Primal Diet, Cave Man Diet, Stone Age Diet, Hunter-Gatherer Diet, the Paleo Diet TM, and a few more names have been used to describe the Paleolithic way of eating. It consists mostly of a low-carb diet that attempts to replicate what our forefathers ate before to the advent of agriculture and the other changes that have occurred in our diets.

Individuals who strive to eat in the manner of our "basic" forefathers face a number of obstacles, as with many other alternative eating methods. So what holds true are the basic principles that most Paleolithic eaters agree on.

Here are some important tips to follow whether you fully embrace this way of eating by going "clean and simple" or ease your way into it gradually.

What foods are considered "forbidden"?

Sugars that have been refined: All sugars should be avoided. White sugar, high fructose corn syrup, confectionery, milk chocolate, pop, and sugar substitutes are all examples. Some Paleolithic advocates allow small amounts of raw honey, unprocessed maple syrup, and coconut sugar as a delicacy, but only on occasion.

Wheat, rye, grain, rice, oats, and maize are just a few of the grains to avoid. Bread, pasta, prepared foods, hotcakes, rolls, biscuits, bagels, and grains are all examples of food diversity. Grains are calorie-dense and contain a lot of starch. Beans, peas, lentils, soybeans, tofu, soy products, and peanuts are all included in the legumes category.

Avoid dairy products such as regular milk, spread, cream, organic product yogurts, frozen yogurt, and processed cheeses.

Some Paleolithic eaters do not consume dairy, whereas others do. Start with refined margarine, Greek yogurt (not natural product seasoned), kefir, coagulated milks, and aged cheeses to relish it every now and then. Lactose (milk sugar) levels are drastically reduced in these matured foods.

Following that would be unprocessed, high-fat dairy products such as crude margarine and cream, which are rich in dissolved fat. The bulk of these are lactose and casein-free and should be sourced from grass-fed, field-raised animals. Milk that has been homogenized or filtered should be avoided at all costs. If you must have it, make sure it is organic, chemical-free, and anti-toxin-free milk. Consider substituting unsweetened almond milk and coconut milk for cow's milk, as nuts are acceptable.

Every now and again, grass-fed margarine is acceptable. If you're going to have cheddar every now and then, make sure it's matured, since ageing reduces the lactose and casein levels dramatically.

Handled meats, such as franks, bologna, and lunchmeats, should be avoided at all costs. If you're going to consume bacon or a hotdog, be sure they don't contain nitrates or nitrites. The bacon debate continues to rage among Paleo enthusiasts, however others believe it is OK provided nitrite/nitrate-free bacon is used, as well as bacon that is devoid of sugar. Others acknowledge that it isn't permissible due to the fact that it is eased. IT'S UP TO YOU!

Shortening, margarines, canola oil, soybean oil, cottonseed oil, nut oil, maize oil, and sunflower oil are all examples of "slightly hydrogenated" oils to avoid. Make sure you examine the mark on your mayonnaise thoroughly.

What are the permitted foods?

Meat, fish, and eggs: Meat, fish, and eggs are perhaps the most important components of the Paleolithic diet. Hamburger, hog, sheep, buffalo, chicken, shrimp, crab, trout, salmon, and mackerel, as well as other wild-caught fish such as sardines, shellfish, mussels, and mollusks, are among them. Bacon and sausage are now again hotly disputed, therefore you must determine whether or not they are healthy. Vegetables: Vegetables are very nutrient-dense and may be consumed in almost unlimited quantities.

Concentrate on various leafy greens. At this stage, opinions vary on whether or not you should remember to consume potatoes and other boring tubers as part of your regular diet. Fruits: Fruits are allowed, but they should be consumed in moderation, especially if you are trying to lose weight.

Natural goods with a lot of sugar, such as dried foods from the ground, should be consumed in moderation.

Nuts and seeds are generally allowed. Because they're heavy in fat, keep your admissions to a minimum to stay in better shape. Macadamias, Brazil nuts, hazelnuts, pistachios, walnuts, almonds, pecans, cashews, squash seeds, sunflower seeds, and pumpkin seeds are just a few of the nuts and seeds available. Peanuts are not permitted since they are considered vegetables.

Olive oil and nut oils, such as coconut oil, are generally considered to be healthy fats. The list of permitted fats includes margarine, palm oil, ghee, and beast fats.

Water is perfect and should be your primary beverage, according to all spokespersons. Tea is generally seen as acceptable, but espresso and alcohol continue to be available in a variety of forms.

Sugar-free or sugar-fortified beverages are not recommended.

I've tried to steer you toward this eating philosophy throughout this collection of plans (and the others in my series). The goal is to gradually change your eating habits without making you feel like there is just one right way to do things. Simply be aware of your grades and make the best decision possible.

Don't be concerned if you can't afford to buy natural or grass-fed beef. Simply buy the necessary ingredients and follow the Paleolithic diet principles. I'd like to think you're involved with this collection of Paleolithic schemes. They're among my family's absolute favorites, and I'm hoping they'll be among yours as well!

DISHES WITH FRITTAS AND EGG

Frittata with a Garden Flavour

Frittatas are a delicious way to start the day. A frittata is a large, flat Italian omelet cooked under the broiler. A large group of people is fed frittatas (5-8). They're also excellent for quick snacks and extras.

Ingredients:

14 cup almond milk (eight eggs)

to taste with salt and pepper

olive oil, 2 tablespoons

2–3 garlic cloves, sliced or smashed finely

2 cups chopped or shredded spinach for kids

12 cup fresh mushrooms, sliced 1 red bell pepper, cut or chunked 1 red onion, chopped

if preferred, 2 tblsp. fresh parsley

Preheat the oven to 425 degrees Fahrenheit for the broiler.

Combine the eggs with the almond milk in a separate dish.

Set aside after mixing well.

Pour the olive oil into a medium-sized stove-safe skillet set over medium heat.

Place the garlic, spinach, red onion, fresh mushrooms, and red ringer pepper in the pan when the oil has warmed up. 6. Cook until the veggies are soft, about 3-4 minutes. 7. Add the egg/almond mixture to the veggies in the pan one at a time.

Reduce the heat to a minimum in the skillet.

Cook for around 10 minutes at a low heat.

Place the stove-safe skillet in the preheated oven once the edges seem to be hard.

Cook for 15-20 minutes at 425°F on a stovetop.

When the center of the frittata is solid and no longer jiggles, the frittata is done.

Cut the frittata into wedges and serve with fresh parsley on top.

Enjoy while it's hot!

Frittata with Veggies

This deliciously crunchy egg dish is a fantastic all-around supper. It's a tempting choice for breakfast because of the wonderful array of veggies.

1 cup chopped broccoli florets

12 c. red onion, chopped

1 pound chopped summer squash

1 cup chopped cooked meat

12 cup chopped sun-dried tomatoes 7 eggs

to taste with salt and pepper

For cooking, coconut oil

Directions:

Preheat the oven to 375 degrees Fahrenheit for the broiler.

liquefy enough coconut oil to coat the bottom of a 10-inch stove-resistant skillet.

Cook until the onions are transparent, then add the broccoli and onions to the griddle.

Cook until the squash is soft, then add the pork and sun dried tomatoes.

Now evenly distribute the mixture on the griddle's lowest portion.

Whisk the eggs in a bowl until well combined, then pour over the mixture in the browning pan.

Cook until the eggs firm up around the pan's edge over medium low heat.

Cook for 10 to 12 minutes on a hot griddle.

When the middle of the frittata is solid, it's ready.

Frittata from Mexico

With your eggs, add a dash of zest and vigor. This tasty meal is perfect for any occasion.

Ingredients:

coconut oil (1 tablespoon)

14 cup chopped onion

1 jalapeo pepper, seeded and sliced

ground beef, 1 pound

1 c. sweet potato, coarsely ground

2 finely minced garlic cloves

stew powder, 1 tbsp

cumin powder (1 teaspoon)

12 cup salsa (without the sugar)

12 eggs are required

to taste with salt and pepper

Preheat your oven to 350 degrees Fahrenheit (180 degrees Celsius).

Sauté the onions and jalapeño in the coconut oil on a large griddle until the onions are soft.

Cook for a few minutes, until the ground hamburger begins to brown.

In a singing pan, add the potato and garlic.

Cook until the yam is tender and the beef is completely carmelized.

Combine the stew powder, cumin, and salsa in a bowl and stir to combine.

In a large mixing bowl, combine the flavors, salsa, and spiciness.

Season with salt and pepper to taste at this time.

Remove the beef mixture from the heat and place it in a glass baking dish about 11" 7" in diameter.

Distribute the meat mixture evenly over the glass pan's bottom half.

Tear open the eggs in a separate mixing dish and thoroughly whisk them together.

In a baking dish, crack the eggs over the meat mixture.

Wrap aluminum foil around the glass skillet.

Cook for 30 minutes under the broiler at 350°F.

Remove the foil after 30 minutes and cook for a further 10-15 minutes, or until the eggs are set in the middle when wiggled.

Remove from the broiler after immovability has been achieved and let cool for a few minutes.

Enjoy by slicing the cake into serving portions.

Quiché

Cups

Solid crustless quiche may now be enjoyed on a regular basis. These morning meal cups may also be stored in the refrigerator until they're ready to reheat and enjoy.

Ingredients:

Meat: 12 pound (ground pork or turkey works well)

1 cup of your favorite vegetables: chile peppers, sliced spinach, scallions or onions, fresh mushrooms

13 cup crumbled cheddar (to taste). (Matured cheese is preferred.)

5 eggs are required

a third of a cup of coconut or almond milk

Directions:

Preheat the oven to 325 degrees Fahrenheit and preheat the broiler.

Using olive oil, grease a biscuit pan.

Prepare your selected meat and, if necessary, channel it.

Then, until the veggies are soft, sauté them.

In a mixing dish, combine the sautéed veggies with the cheddar. Set aside right now.

In a lubed biscuit tin, whisk together the eggs and milk, then pour in equal amounts of hitter.

Fill each biscuit cup with desired amount of meat and veggie/cheddar mix.

Preheat oven to 350°F and bake for 20-25 minutes, until golden brown.

Allow to cool for a minute.

Take biscuits out of the platter and eat them.

Eggs with Turkey

Perfectly cooked eggs and spicy ground turkey burgers. It's one-of-a-kind, full, and tasty.

Ingredients:

12 lb. turkey ground

3 tbsp. onions, coarsely chopped

coconut aminos, 2 tblsp.

cayenne pepper (12 tsp.)

12 tsp powdered garlic

1 tsp. sea salt 1 tsp. cayenne

For frying, use coconut oil or water.

A total of four eggs

Mix the turkey, onions, aminos, cayenne pepper, garlic powder, salt, and pepper together in a large mixing basin.

Combine all of the ingredients in a large mixing bowl.

Make four patties using this mixture.

Place a large skillet over medium heat with just enough coconut oil or splash to coat the bottom of the pan.

In a searing pan, place the four patties.

Cook the patties for around 5 minutes before flipping them.

Cook for a further 5 minutes, or until the patties are fully cooked.

Set aside this container or remove the patties so you may go on to the following stage with a similar potential.

Carefully break each egg in turn on a preheated griddle, making every effort to retain the egg in its original form. When your food is hot, this technique is most effective.

Cook for 3-5 minutes, or until the egg whites are no longer runny, covered in the skillet.

When the eggs are done, remove them from the pan and place one on top of each beef patty.

As desired, season with salt and pepper.

Chili

Crepes A twist on traditional crepes with tomfoolery and filling This egg wrap-up is memorable because of the ground beef and spicy chopped vegetables.

Ingredients:

14 cup water 14 cup onions, mushrooms, red and green peppers, divided

For cooking, dice these.

lean ground beef, 1 pound

14 teaspoon garlic powder 12 teaspoon salt

12 tsp. powdered stew

112 tsp coconut aminos

pepper, black

3 tablespoons diced green onions

Crepe

eggs (three)

14 cup flour made from coconut

12 cup coconut or almond milk

a quarter cup of water, a pinch of salt

Directions:

Add the water, onions, mushrooms, red and green peppers, and salt & pepper to taste to a large, preheated pan.

Heat on high for 7–8 minutes, or until onions are soft.

Separate the meat from the vegetables and add it to the mixture.

Combine the salt, garlic powder, bean stew powder, aminos, and dark pepper in a large mixing bowl.

Continue to cook the beef over medium heat, stirring occasionally, until it is fully done.

Set aside the hamburger mixture in a basin.

It's time to get your crepes started.

In a large mixing basin, combine the ingredients for the crepes.

As you combine the ingredients together, be sure to separate any lumps of flour.

Preheat your oven to its highest setting and lightly oil a skillet.

Pour approximately a quarter cup of the crepe batter into your container and swirl it around to evenly coat the pan.

Heat till you see small air pockets appearing all over the place on medium-high heat.

crepe.

The crepe's sides should turn a brilliant brown color as well.

Carefully remove the crepe from the container with a delicate spatula and place it on a plate large enough to accommodate it.

By placing the meat mixture in the center of the crepe, you can fill it with it.

Green onions should be sprinkled over the meat mixture.

As you get the sides into the middle, fold one end over the combination and begin moving.

With fresh fruit on the side

Omelet with roasted red peppers and arugula

This dish's wonderful mix of flavors reflects the dish's beautiful difference.

Ingredients:

For cooking, coconut oil

1 cup hacked arugula 1 onion, sliced 1 pepper, chopped

4 eggs (beaten) 1 tomato, chopped

to taste with salt and pepper

1 lemon, squeezed

Directions:

Place a small amount of coconut oil in a griddle and heat over medium-high heat.

When the oil is hot, add the chopped onions and cook until they are translucent.

Then add the cleaved chime peppers and cook until soft.

Blend in the arugula and tomato slices until everything is well combined.

Cook for about three minutes with the ingredients.

Pour in the fried eggs and continue to mix well until they are thoroughly cooked.

Place on a plate after removing the container.

If you want to be extra fancy, drizzle some fresh lemon juice on top.

Frittata à la B.B.C.

It's impossible to beat the perfect combination of bacon and broccoli. While bacon is still a Paleo staple, you get to decide whether or not this diet is right for you. If you can handle dairy, the addition of matured destroyed cheddar rounds it out.

12 pound cooked and crumbled bacon (nitrite/nitrate) free)

broccoli tail 1 (florets just, broken into little pieces)

A total of eight eggs

a total of 112 quarts of coconut milk

1 tbsp. melted ghee/spread

12 cup aged cheese that has been destroyed

to taste with salt and pepper

For cooking, coconut oil

Preheat the oven to 425 degrees Fahrenheit for the broiler. (A skillet that can go in the oven is required for this recipe.)

Cook bacon on a griddle or in the microwave until it reaches the desired level of freshness.

Cut the broccoli florets off the top and soften them for 4 to 5 minutes in a microwave dish or over a pot of boiling water.

Mix the eggs, coconut milk, spread, salt, and pepper together in a separate bowl.

Combine the broccoli and crumbled bacon in a large mixing bowl.

Pour the mixture into a skillet with a small amount of space in it.

It dissolved a large amount of coconut oil.

Cook until the frittata's sides begin to firm up, about 10 minutes on medium heat.

Remove the frittata from the heat and top it with the crumbled cheddar cheese (optional).

In a preheated oven, place the entire skillet.

Cook until the frittata's focal point is firm, about 15-20 minutes.

Allow 5 to 10 minutes to cool after removing from the stove.

12. Enjoy by slicing into wedges.

Casserole de Petits-Dejeuners Savory

To start your day, try this quick and filling dish. This meal is simple to prepare thanks to the cooked meat and fresh vegetables.

Ingredients:

6 eggs are required.

14 pound cooked meat

14 cup mushrooms, fresh cut

3 tblsp. onions, chopped

1 tsp. salt and pepper for each person

12 tsp powdered garlic

paprika (12 tbsp.)

12 tsp. thyme (dried)

For fixing, use aged, smashed cheddar (optional)

Preheat your oven to 350 degrees Fahrenheit (180 degrees Celsius).

Combine all of the ingredients in a large mixing bowl, except for the cheddar that will be used as a garnish, and blend until smooth.

Fill an 8" x 8" baking dish halfway with the mixture.

strew crumbled cheddar across the player's highest point (optional).

Cook for 45 minutes in a preheated broiler.

Serve immediately after slicing

Casserole de Zucchini y Pork

Chapter Two

Eggs with Turkey

Perfectly cooked eggs and spicy ground turkey burgers. It's one-of-a-kind, full, and tasty.

Ingredients:

12 lb. turkey ground

3 tbsp. onions, coarsely chopped

coconut aminos, 2 tblsp.

cayenne pepper (12 tsp.)

12 tsp powdered garlic

1 tsp. sea salt 1 tsp. cayenne

For frying, use coconut oil or water.

A total of four eggs

Mix the turkey, onions, aminos, cayenne pepper, garlic powder, salt, and pepper together in a large mixing basin.

Combine all of the ingredients in a large mixing bowl.

Make four patties using this mixture.

Place a large skillet over medium heat with just enough coconut oil or splash to coat the bottom of the pan.

In a searing pan, place the four patties.

Cook the patties for around 5 minutes before flipping them.

Cook for a further 5 minutes, or until the patties are fully cooked.

Set aside this container or remove the patties so you may go on to the following stage with a similar potential.

Carefully break each egg in turn on a preheated griddle, making every effort to retain the egg in its original form. When your food is hot, this technique is most effective.

Cook for 3-5 minutes, or until the egg whites are no longer runny, covered in the skillet.

When the eggs are done, remove them from the pan and place one on top of each beef patty.

As desired, season with salt and pepper.

Chili

Crepes A twist on traditional crepes with tomfoolery and filling This egg wrap-up is memorable because of the ground beef and spicy chopped vegetables.

Ingredients:

14 cup water 14 cup onions, mushrooms, red and green peppers, divided

For cooking, dice these.

lean ground beef, 1 pound

14 teaspoon garlic powder 12 teaspoon salt

12 tsp. powdered stew

112 tsp coconut aminos

pepper, black

3 tablespoons diced green onions

Crepe

eggs (three)

14 cup flour made from coconut

12 cup coconut or almond milk

a quarter cup of water, a pinch of salt

Directions:

Add the water, onions, mushrooms, red and green peppers, and salt & pepper to taste to a large, preheated pan.

Heat on high for 7–8 minutes, or until onions are soft.

Separate the meat from the vegetables and add it to the mixture.

Combine the salt, garlic powder, bean stew powder, aminos, and dark pepper in a large mixing bowl.

Continue to cook the beef over medium heat, stirring occasionally, until it is fully done.

Set aside the hamburger mixture in a basin.

It's time to get your crepes started.

In a large mixing basin, combine the ingredients for the crepes.

As you combine the ingredients together, be sure to separate any lumps of flour.

Preheat your oven to its highest setting and lightly oil a skillet.

Pour approximately a quarter cup of the crepe batter into your container and swirl it around to evenly coat the pan.

Heat till you see small air pockets appearing all over the place on medium-high heat.

crepe.

The crepe's sides should turn a brilliant brown color as well.

Carefully remove the crepe from the container with a delicate spatula and place it on a plate large enough to accommodate it.

By placing the meat mixture in the center of the crepe, you can fill it with it.

Green onions should be sprinkled over the meat mixture.

As you get the sides into the middle, fold one end over the combination and begin moving.

With fresh fruit on the side

Omelet with roasted red peppers and arugula

This dish's wonderful mix of flavors reflects the dish's beautiful difference.

Ingredients:

For cooking, coconut oil

1 cup hacked arugula 1 onion, sliced 1 pepper, chopped

4 eggs (beaten) 1 tomato, chopped

to taste with salt and pepper

1 lemon, squeezed

Directions:

Place a small amount of coconut oil in a griddle and heat over medium-high heat.

When the oil is hot, add the chopped onions and cook until they are translucent.

Then add the cleaved chime peppers and cook until soft.

Blend in the arugula and tomato slices until everything is well combined.

Cook for about three minutes with the ingredients.

Pour in the fried eggs and continue to mix well until they are thoroughly cooked.

Place on a plate after removing the container.

If you want to be extra fancy, drizzle some fresh lemon juice on top.

Frittata à la B.B.C.

It's impossible to beat the perfect combination of bacon and broccoli. While bacon is still a Paleo staple, you get to decide whether or not this diet is right for you. If you can handle dairy, the addition of matured destroyed cheddar rounds it out.

12 pound cooked and crumbled bacon (nitrite/nitrate) free)

broccoli tail 1 (florets just, broken into little pieces)

A total of eight eggs

a total of 112 quarts of coconut milk

1 tbsp. melted ghee/spread

12 cup aged cheese that has been destroyed

to taste with salt and pepper

For cooking, coconut oil

Preheat the oven to 425 degrees Fahrenheit for the broiler. (A skillet that can go in the oven is required for this recipe.)

Cook bacon on a griddle or in the microwave until it reaches the desired level of freshness.

Cut the broccoli florets off the top and soften them for 4 to 5 minutes in a microwave dish or over a pot of boiling water.

Mix the eggs, coconut milk, spread, salt, and pepper together in a separate bowl.

Combine the broccoli and crumbled bacon in a large mixing bowl.

Pour the mixture into a skillet with a small amount of space in it.

It dissolved a large amount of coconut oil.

Cook until the frittata's sides begin to firm up, about 10 minutes on medium heat.

Remove the frittata from the heat and top it with the crumbled cheddar cheese (optional).

In a preheated oven, place the entire skillet.

Cook until the frittata's focal point is firm, about 15-20 minutes.

Allow 5 to 10 minutes to cool after removing from the stove.
12. Enjoy by slicing into wedges.

Casserole de Petits-Dejeuners Savory

To start your day, try this quick and filling dish. This meal is simple to prepare thanks to the cooked meat and fresh vegetables.

Ingredients:

6 eggs are required.

14 pound cooked meat

14 cup mushrooms, fresh cut

3 tblsp. onions, chopped

1 tsp. salt and pepper for each person

12 tsp powdered garlic

paprika (12 tbsp.)

12 tsp. thyme (dried)

For fixing, use aged, smashed cheddar (optional)

Preheat your oven to 350 degrees Fahrenheit (180 degrees Celsius).

Combine all of the ingredients in a large mixing bowl, except for the cheddar that will be used as a garnish, and blend until smooth.

Fill an 8" x 8" baking dish halfway with the mixture.

strew crumbled cheddar across the player's highest point (optional).

Cook for 45 minutes in a preheated broiler.

Serve immediately after slicing

Casserole de Zucchini y Pork

Chapter Three

Casserole de Zucchini y Pork

This generous and scrumptious dish, which is part goulash and part frittata, is hearty and filling without being heavy.

Ingredients:

a chopped red onion

4 finely minced garlic cloves

A total of eight eggs

2 c. ruined pork

1 shredded zucchini

2 tsp basil (fresh)

to taste with salt and pepper

12 - 1 cup matured cheddar cheese that has been ruined (optional)

Preheat the oven to 350 degrees Fahrenheit and prepare the dish.

In a skillet, caramelize your onion and garlic over medium heat.

Allow the onion to stay in the pan after the heat has been turned off.

Combine the eggs, pork, zucchini, basil, salt, and pepper in a blender bowl and blend until smooth.

Stir in the onions and garlic that have been sautéed.

Empty the mixture into a greased 9" x 13" baking dish and evenly distribute it.

If desired, finish with crumbled cheddar.

Cook for 30 minutes on the stove. To see if it's done, look in the middle.

Put the dish under the grill for 4 to 5 minutes if you want to sauté the top. 10. Serve immediately after cutting.

BREAD AND MUFFINS

Egg Cups for Breakfast

This versatile dish is ideal for a quick breakfast, a delectable early lunch, or a substantial canapé. Extra meat from the previous evening's supper can be used in this simple and quick meal. Egg cups that aren't used right away can be refrigerated and served later.

Ingredients:

1 tsp olive oil OR 1 tsp olive oil spray

2 cups cooked cubes of meat

12 eggs are required

to taste with salt and pepper

14 cup aged cheddar cheese, crumbled (discretionary assuming that you eat dairy)

3 tbsp. chives (cut)

Preheat the oven to 350 degrees Fahrenheit and prepare the dish.

Wipe or lightly spray each biscuit cup with olive oil.

In the lower part of each cup, place a couple of meat solid shapes.

Allow an egg to fall onto the meat after cracking it.

Repeat this process until you've filled all of your biscuit cups with an egg.

To taste, season each egg cup with a pinch of sea salt and black pepper.

If desired, garnish each egg with a small amount of crumbled cheddar and chopped chives.

Bake for 20 minutes, or until the eggs are cooked through.

Take the biscuit cups out of the oven and serve them warm.

Almond Bread with Cranberries

This bread is made soggy with zucchini as a fixing and is made hearty with the addition of almond supper and spread. Cranberries, raw honey, nuts, and other flavors infuse this delectable bread with flavor.

4 eggs (optional)

2 zucchinis, peeled and grated

a quarter-cup of almond butter

1 cup cranberries, dried but not sweetened

1 pound of almond flour

2 tsp honey (raw)

Cinnamon, 112 teaspoons

nutmeg (112 tsp.)

1 teaspoon spice blend for pumpkin pie

baking soda (1 teaspoon)

14 tsp. sea salt 14 tsp. clove powder

34 cup walnuts cleaved

Preheat the oven to 350 degrees Fahrenheit and prepare the dish.

Use an olive oil shower or a paper towel to coat a 9" x 5" portion container in olive oil.

Separate the egg yolks and whites into two bowls.

Egg yolks should be thoroughly beaten.

Except for the walnuts, combine all of the remaining ingredients with the egg yolks.

Each of the ingredients should be thoroughly combined.

Using an electric mixer, whip the egg whites until they form solid peaks in a separate bowl.

With the egg/zucchini mixture, gently fold in the egg whites. 9. Stir in the hacked walnuts until they are evenly distributed.

Fill a lubed portion pan halfway with the hitter.

Bake for an hour, or until golden brown on top. 12. Insert a toothpick or a cake analyzer into the center of the bread to check for doneness. When only a few pieces are visible on a toothpick or a tester, it's done.

Before removing the bread from the pan, let it cool for 15-20 minutes.

Cut to desired thickness once it has cooled, and enjoy.

Muffins made with pumpkin and gingerbread

These clammy, delectable wheat-free biscuits evoke warm gingerbread cookies.

Ingredients:

12 CUP CONTAINED COCONUT FAT

cinnamon, 2 tsp.

12 tsp. nutmeg, powdered

12 tsp ginger, powdered

14 tsp. cloves (ground)

12 tsp sodium bicarbonate

12 tsp powdered baking

12 tsp sodium

1 can of soup Pumpkin pureed to the nth degree.

A total of four eggs

14 cup crude honey or unprocessed maple syrup 2-3 tablespoons olive oil

1 tbsp vanilla extract (unadulterated)

Garnish with pecans or pumpkin seeds (optional)

Preheat the oven to 400 degrees Fahrenheit for the broiler.

Using coconut oil or olive oil spray, lightly grease your biscuit skillet.

Combine the flour, spices, pop, baking powder, and salt in a medium-sized mixing bowl.

Pour the pureed pumpkin into another bowl.

Each egg should be added one at a time, blending thoroughly after each addition. 6. In a blender, combine the olive oil, honey, and vanilla until smooth. 7. Mix the flour and pumpkin together with a mixer until most of the irregularities are gone. 8. Using a large spoon, scoop equal amounts of dough into your prepared biscuit dish, filling each biscuit about two-thirds full. 9. If desired, a few seeds or pecans can be sprinkled on the highest point of each biscuit.

10. 20 minutes, or until an analyzer inserted into the center of a biscuit yields only scraps rather than liquid batter.

Allow for a few moments of resting time before transferring the biscuits to a wire rack to cool.

Banana Almond Bread is a delicious bread made with almonds and bananas.

A thick, soggy bread that's perfect for breakfast or as a late-night snack. Coconut, cacao powder, and pumpkin are twirled into the mixture.

Ingredients:

1 cup apricot jam

1 cup coconut husks (unsweetened)

2 bananas (medium)

2 quail

1 tbsp flour

baking soda (1 teaspoon)

14 cup pumpkin puree (from a can)

3 tbsp cacao powder (not sweetened)

if desired, 1 tablespoon honey

Directions:

Preheat the oven to 350 degrees Fahrenheit (180 degrees Celsius).

Combine the almond butter, coconut, bananas, eggs, baking powder, and pop in a blender bowl. Make sure the bananas are well crushed so that the batter holds together.

Fill a lubed portion pan with this mixture.

Toss the pumpkin, cacao powder, and honey together in a separate bowl.

Pour this mixture down the center of the banana batter hitter in the portion skillet and twirl it into the batter with a blade.

Place the portion container on the preheated stove for 40 minutes. When you shake the container, the middle should be firm, and only a few morsels should be embedded and removed on a toothpick or cake analyzer.

Before transferring the bread to a cooling rack, allow it to cool slightly.

Cut to desired thickness once it has cooled.

Sweet Buns with Cinnamon

These cinnamon buns are delicious when they're hot off the stove.

Ingredients:

14 teaspoon baking soda, 2-3 tablespoons coconut flour

14 teaspoon cinnamon 1/8 teaspoon sea salt

Nutmeg, a pinch

1/8 tsp almond extract (unadulterated)

1 ovary

almond or coconut milk, 2 tblsp

1 to 2 tablespoons extra virgin olive oil

1 teaspoon honey (raw)

1 to 112 cup dried fruit, slashed

Preheat the oven to 375 degrees Fahrenheit for the broiler.

In a small mixing bowl, whisk together the coconut flour, baking soda, salt, cinnamon, and nutmeg.

Make a thorough mixture.

In the center of the mixture, create a well.

In the well, mix together the almond extract, egg, milk, oil, and honey.

With a fork, thoroughly combine the ingredients, removing as many lumps as possible.

Allow for a two- or three-minute rest period to allow the coconut flour to absorb the liquid.

Place the batter on a baking sheet that has been lined with material.

Form the hitter into a 12-inch thick rectangle on the material-lined baking sheet.

Sprinkle cinnamon on top of the dried organic product.

Roll up your organic product hitter like a cinnamon roll using the edge of the material paper.

Bake the roll in the oven for 20-25 minutes, or until golden brown. 13. Remove the broiler pan from the oven and set aside to cool for a few minutes.

14. Enjoy by slicing to the desired thickness.

Muffins with Bananas & Almonds

The nutty combination of almond meal, coconut flour, and almond margarine in the muffins is the perfect complement to the soggy bananas.

14 cup almond meal 12 cup coconut flour

12 tsp powdered baking

14 tsp. bicarbonate of soda

a third of a cup of honey in its natural state

sea salt, a pinch

A total of four eggs

1 tbsp almond butter (for storing)

2 bananas, mashed to perfection

1 tbsp vanilla extract (unadulterated)

1 tsp. coconut or olive oil

Preheat the oven to 375 degrees Fahrenheit for the broiler.

Combine the flour, almond meal, baking powder, baking soda, honey, and salt in a large mixing bowl.

Combine the eggs, almond butter, bananas, vanilla extract, and oil in a separate bowl.

Slowly pour the dry ingredients into the mixing bowl with the wet ingredients, stirring constantly until the batter is uniform in appearance. 5. Divide the player evenly between the biscuit tins that have been lightly lubed. 6. Cook for 20 to 25 minutes on a preheated stove.

When the biscuits are done, remove them from the broiler and set them aside in the pan to cool for a few minutes.

Place the biscuits on a cooling rack to cool before serving.

PANCAKES AND WAFFLES are two of the most popular breakfast foods in the United States.

Chapter Four

Pancakes made with Coconut Flour

Coconut flour is used in these wheat flour alternative hotcakes.

Add a garnish of your favorite organic product or nut butter to finish.

3 room-temperature eggs are required.

1 tbsp vanilla extract (unadulterated)

coconut milk, 1/2 gallon

1/2 tsp baking soda 1/4 tsp sea salt

coconut flour, 1/3 cup

Whip the eggs until frothy in a mixing bowl using a hand blender.

Do this for two minutes at the most.

Blend the eggs with the vanilla extract and milk until smooth.

Combine the salt, pop, and flour in a separate bowl and thoroughly mix them together.

Pour the flour mixture into the eggs and whisk them together thoroughly.

Spot an iron over medium heat with a light coating of coconut oil.

Pour a small amount of player into the hot frying pan and spread it out with the back of a spoon.

Cook until bubbles appear in the center and around the edges of the flapjack.

Cook until the hotcake is browned on the other side, gently flipping it over.

Add your favorite toppings to the top.

Waffles de Liberté

Gluten-free, grain-free, and dairy-free waffles are a delicious treat. Spread almond butter on the waffles and top with fresh strawberries, blackberries, or blueberries.

Ingredients:

2 enormous ovaries

14 cup coconut milk or almond milk

a total of 12 cup almond flour

1 tbsp. baking soda, 1 tbsp. sea salt

cinnamon, a pinch

Directions:

Preheat the waffle iron to the temperature that you prefer.

To make the froth, whisk together the eggs and milk. A hand blender, you may notice, makes this process easier.

Put all of the extra dry fixings in a separate bowl and thoroughly mix them together.

Blend the egg/milk mixture until smooth in the mixing bowl with the combined dry ingredients.

In a preheated waffle iron, pour 1/4 cup of the player.

Remove after cooking until golden brown.

Add a new product of your choice, as well as almond spread, to the top. Yum!

Pancakes filled with nuts

These hotcakes are hearty and delicious without the wheat. These pancakes have a warm, nutty flavor thanks to the chestnut flour and almond dinner.

1 cup flour de châtaignier de châtaignier de châ

12 cup ground almonds

a third of a cup of almond or coconut milk

1 teaspoon honey (raw) (optional)

2 whites from 2 eggs

For cooking, coconut oil

Directions:

In a large mixing bowl, whisk together the flour, almond meal, milk, and honey.

Hand-blender the egg whites until they form solid pinnacles in a separate bowl.

Fold the egg whites into the batter with a gentle crease.

In a griddle, heat a small amount of coconut oil over medium-high heat.

When the skillet is hot, add about two tablespoons of batter, or more if you prefer thicker pancakes.

Allow 2 to 3 minutes for little air pockets to form and the sides to solidify slightly before flipping.

Remove from the broiling pan once the next side is a brilliant brown color.

Serve with your favorite toppings, such as pure maple syrup and berries, while they're still warm.

Coconut Pancakes with a Fluffy Fluffy Fluffy Fluffy Fluffy Fluffy

These fluffy hotcakes are charmingly tall. They're difficult to resist when drizzled with pure maple syrup or topped with strawberries.

Ingredients:

4 chilled eggs

coconut milk (1 cup)

2 tsp vanilla extract, pure and unadulterated

1 teaspoon honey (raw) (optional)

12 CUP CONTAINED COCONUT FAT

baking soda (1 teaspoon)

12 tsp. salt from the sea

For cooking, coconut oil

Whisk the eggs until frothy in a mixing bowl. It's possible that a hand mixer will be necessary.

In a large mixing bowl, combine the eggs, milk, vanilla, and honey.

Combine flour, pop, and salt in a separate bowl and thoroughly combine.

Heat a skillet or frying pan over medium heat with just enough coconut oil to cover the bottom.

Pour or spoon enough batter to shape your pancake once the oil has warmed up.

Cook until the edges of the flapjack dry out and solidify, and bubbles form throughout the pancake.

Cook until golden brown on the other side of the hotcake.

Using your favorite garnish, such as berries and pure maple syrup, top your flapjack.

Latkes made from sweet potato

Latkes are traditionally made by grinding raw potatoes, usually russets, which have a high starch content. The latkes are seared in warmed oil until they are a brilliant brown color on both sides after they have been shaped. You can avoid the high starch content of potatoes by using yams, while still enjoying a satisfying treat.

Ingredients:

5 c sweet potato, ground

2 quail

2 tbsp. minced onions

cinnamon (1 teaspoon)

to taste with salt and pepper

For cooking, coconut oil

Directions:

In a large blender bowl, combine all of the ingredients.

To soften a spoonful of coconut oil, heat an iron or griddle over medium heat.

Take a small amount of the potato mixture and shape it into little cakes in a hot frying pan or skillet.

Cook for 3-5 minutes on each side, or until golden brown and fully warmed.

On the off chance that you want, top the latkes with delicacies like fried eggs and bacon.

Pancakes made with apples and cinnamon

These hotcakes have an energizing poignancy thanks to the green apples. You'll notice that they're both tasty and satisfying.

Ingredients:

12 cup ground almonds

12 cup sliced and grated green apple

a quarter of an egg white

¼ cup crude honey or coconut sugar

¼ cup almond milk, coconut milk, or water

1 tablespoon new lemon juice

12 tsp sodium bicarbonate

¼ teaspoon cinnamon

¼ teaspoon salt

Directions:\sIn an enormous bowl, join every one of the fixings until they are all around mixed and are the consistency of a pourable batter.

Set the hitter to the side while you heat your skillet on the stovetop.

Spray your griddle with olive oil cooking shower or coconut oil.

Spoon 1/4 cup of the flapjack player into the skillet and cook on medium-high for 5 minutes on each side.

Remove from the dish and eat!

Chapter Five

GRAIN-FREE CEREALS

C oconut Blackberry Bars

Prepackaged café fail to measure up to these new and fruity breakfast bars.

Ingredients:\s1 cup almond flour\s½ cup unsweetened destroyed coconut

cinnamon (1 teaspoon)

1 tbsp flour

12 tsp sodium bicarbonate

12 tsp. salt from the sea

¼ cup crude honey

2 ready bananas, mashed

2 quail

2 tablespoons softened coconut oil or olive oil

1 tbsp vanilla extract (unadulterated)

a third of a cup of coconut or almond milk

1 cup blackberries, new or thawed

Preheat the oven to 350 degrees Fahrenheit and prepare the dish.

Prepare an 8" × 8" baking container with coconut splash or olive oil splash and set aside.

Using a huge bowl, combine as one the flour, destroyed coconut, cinnamon, baking powder, pop, and salt. 4. Add the honey to this combination and blend.

Now include the bananas, eggs, oil, vanilla, and 1/4 cup of almond milk.

Mix completely until every one of the fixings are moist. 7. Be certain the player has the consistency of a treat hitter. In the event that essential, add extra measures of almond milk to accomplish this.

Gently overlap in the blackberries, being mindful so as not to destroy them too much.

Spoon the player into the lubed baking pan.

Bake for around 40 minutes or until the hitter is brilliant brown along the sides.

Remove skillet from the broiler and permit the bars to cool before slicing.

Granola Crunch with Chocolate

You've come to the right place if you're looking for a modest handful of crunch. For an energy boost or a late-night snack, this is a must-try.

Ingredients:

12 cup sunflower seeds in their natural state

12 cup pumpkin seeds in their natural state

1 pound of almond flour

1 cup coconut husks (unsweetened)

2 cups sliced or chopped raw almonds

2 tbsp cacao powder (not sweetened)

1 tsp cinnamon powder

12 CUP COCONUT OLIVE

12 c. honey (raw)

1 tbsp vanilla essence (unadulterated)

Preheat oven to 325°F.

Using gently oiled aluminum foil, line a cookie sheet with treats.

Toss the sunflower seeds, pumpkin seeds, almond feast, coconut, almonds, cacao powder, and cinnamon together in a large mixing bowl.

Consolidate any remaining oil, honey, or vanilla in a microwave-safe dish.

Microwave the wet fixings bowl for 20 to 30 seconds on high to warm it up. This will make it easier for your mixture to pour.

Mix the wet and dry ingredients well together.

Ensure that the coating is applied evenly.

Fill your foil-lined cookie with the mixture.

Distribute the treats evenly on the sheet of treats.

Place the treat sheet on the burner for 25 minutes, keeping an eye on the mixture to ensure it doesn't burn. (If you want it to cook evenly, you may need to mix it once throughout the interaction.)

Allow the mash to cool after removing the treat sheet from the broiler. As the mixture cools down, you'll notice it becomes more crunchy.

This formula may be taken straight or mixed with almond milk in place of a grain cereal.

Granola with Cranberry and Nuts

This granola is great for a quick energy boost. You may eat it alone as a snack or make a nutty morning cereal by combining it with coconut or almond milk.

1 cup toasted pecans (recipe below)

1 cup chopped toasted almonds

1 cup cranberries, dry but not sweetened

14 – 12 cup unsweetened crushed coconut 14 teaspoon cinnamon powder

To taste, season with salt

Directions:

In a mixing dish, combine all of the components.

Plan may be eaten as a snack or with a splash of coconut or almond milk.

MORE SMOOTHIES

Smoothie with Banana and Berry

Bananas help smoothies get that thick velvety texture that elevates them to new heights. This morning drink is certain to be a hit thanks to frozen berries and a ginger kick.

1 banana, peeled and sliced

12 c. berries, frozen

coconut water (1 cup)

a peeled and thumbnail-sized chunk of fresh ginger

cinnamon (1 teaspoon)

1 teaspoon honey (raw)

ice (two cups)

Directions:

Fill a blender halfway with all of the ingredients.

Process on high until the mixture reaches a smooth consistency.

Pour the mixture into a large glass and enjoy the burst of energy.

Smoothie with Berries and Nuts

This berry smoothie gets a twist with finely powdered nuts. It's very refreshing, in fact.

Ingredients:

1 cup water or almond or coconut milk

12 c. berries, frozen

walnuts, 14 cup

1 teaspoon honey (raw)

cinnamon (1 teaspoon)

ice, 1 cup

Put all of the ingredients in a blender and mix until smooth.

Process on high until the mixture reaches a smooth consistency.

Enjoy in a large glass.

Sausage Breakfast

If you can freshly grind your own meat, this recipe is a fantastic way to put it to good use.

Ingredients:

2 lb. beef mince

1 lb. pork mince

2 teaspoons fresh thyme 2 teaspoons fresh wise 1 teaspoon fresh rosemary 2 tablespoons sea salt

112 tsp. cayenne

1 tsp nutmeg (freshly ground)

cayenne pepper (12 tsp.)

Instructions: In a large mixing basin, combine all of the ingredients.

1 to 2 creeps in diameter, form the meat mixture into little round balls or connectors.

Use a little amount of coconut oil on the bottom of a griddle or pan on your stove over a medium heat setting.

Cook for 10 to 15 minutes, until the beef adjusts are charred and cooked through.

Remove the meat from the container and pour any excess oil or oil into a separate container. Flapjacks, waffles, and eggs are all better with this.

SALADS

Lobster Salad with Asian Flavors

One of my favorite foods to eat is lobster. I don't always get to enjoy it, but when I do, I like to cook this mixed greens salad. This recipe is also enjoyable since you can wrap the lobster filling within your cabbage leaves (rather than cutting them as the recipe directs) and enjoy them as I have shown in the photograph. It's excellent in either case!

1 pound cooked lobster flesh (about 1 pound)

2 cups Napa cabbage (roughly sliced)

12 red ringer pepper, thinly sliced 8 ounce jar water chestnuts, drained 12 cup fresh parsley, chopped 14 cup toasted fragmented almonds

Dressing:

chicken broth, 2 tbsp

coconut aminos, 2 tblsp.

1 teaspoon of extra virgin olive oil

sesame oil, 1 tblsp.

1 tsp. freshly grated ginger

Cut the lobster flesh into smaller pieces to make it easier to work with.

In a medium mixing basin, toss together the cabbage, chile pepper, water chestnuts, parsley, and almonds.

Thoroughly combine all fixings.

Combine the stock, aminos, olive oil, and salt in a small bowl. ginger, sesame oil

Dress salad with dressing.

Coat with a light tossing.

Salad with warm shrimp

3 lemon juice

1 teaspoon chopped garlic, 3 tablespoons crude honey
to taste with salt and pepper

olive oil, 2 tablespoons

12 pound raw shrimp, washed and stripped

12 cup snap peas, diced 2 medium estimates zucchini, chopped 12 cup broccoli sprouts 14 teaspoon fresh ginger, coarsely grated

2 tbsp sesame seeds, lightly roasted (optional)

Directions:

Combine the lemon juice, honey, garlic, salt, and pepper in a small bowl and whisk to combine.

Allow for a few minutes of marinating time after pouring half of the mixture over the shrimp.

Over medium-high heat, heat the olive oil in a large pan.

When the skillet is heated, add the shrimp and cook until they are pink and fully cooked.

Toss the ginger, snap peas, zucchini, and sprouts together in a medium mixing dish.

In a large mixing bowl, combine the warm, cooked shrimp.

Combine the remaining lemon juice mixture and sesame seeds in a mixing bowl.

Right away, serve.

If you have some fresh pineapple on hand, adding a couple of lumps is a nice variation. It's not necessary, but it adds a whole other level of complexity.

Ingredients in Poached Egg Salad

A total of four eggs

lemon juice, 3 teaspoons

12 teaspoon freshly ground pepper 2 tablespoons Dijon mustard 34 teaspoon sea salt

12 CUP OF OLIVE

lean ground beef (4 ounces)

6 c. greens, combined

4 oz. aged cheddar cheese, crumbled (optional)

Directions

In an egg poacher, a saucepan, or the microwave, poach the eggs.

Cook for 4 minutes in an egg poacher or 2 minutes in the microwave until the whites are set but the yolks are still liquid.

Combine the lemon juice, mustard, salt, and pepper in a blender to create the dressing.

Fill a medium mixing bowl halfway with the dressing and slowly drizzle in the olive oil until it thickens.

Remove the item from circulation.

Cook the beef until it is browned in a pan over medium heat.

Toss the greens with the dressing and toss well.

Ground hamburger and shredded cheese are sprinkled on top.

Last but not least, top each salad dish with one egg.

SOUPS

Soup with Beef and Cabbage

Throughout the year, I like soups, and this one is particularly wonderful and filling. This one is also highly healthy, thanks to all of the fantastic food sources.

Ingredients:

stewing beef (12 pound)

2 inlet leaves and 3 quarts water

a little cabbage head

4 pound carrots, cut 4 pound celery stems, chopped 1 pound onion, diced 15 pound diced tomatoes

8.8 oz. Tomato juice is 100% pure.

Fill a large saucepan with 3 quarts of water and place the hamburger in it.

Add the leaves that are straight.

To guarantee tender meat, cover the saucepan and cook it for 3 hours.

Cabbage, carrots, celery, and onion should all be chopped.

In the same saucepan as the meat, add the veggies. Add 30 minutes to the cooking time.

Remove the straight leaves and combine the tomatoes and tomato juice in a bowl.

Return to a boil before serving.

Note: Tomatoes and tomato juice may be used when other veggies are added if desired.

Soup de pommes de terre

1 tbsp coconut oil 1 tbsp coconut flour

12 cup chicken broth 12 cup sweet potatoes, cooked cubed

14 tsp ginger powder (or new, to taste)

1/8 tsp. cinnamon powder

1/8 tsp. nutmeg, ground

coconut milk (1 cup)

to taste with salt and pepper

Directions:

Cook the coconut flour and coconut oil in a pan over medium-low heat, constantly stirring, until the mixture acquires a light caramel color.

Bring up to a boil the chicken stock.

Reduce the heat to low and add the yams, ginger, cinnamon, and nutmeg after that.

Cook for 5 minutes more on low, stirring often.

Take the mixture out of the saucepan and place it in a blender.

Soup should be pureed.

Now it's time to return to the pot.

Now, gently reheat the soup with the coconut milk. 9. Serve with a pinch of salt and pepper.

Soup with Vegetables is a simple recipe that anybody can make.

14 cup sliced onion 1 cup daintily cut carrots Ingredients: 2 teaspoons coconut oil

1 cup zucchini, finely diced

2 tblsp parsley, fresh

thyme (1/4 teaspoon)

pepper (1/8 teaspoon)

2 c.

Directions:

Heat the coconut oil in a medium-sized saucepan.

Add the onion after it's warmed up and sauté until it's transparent.

In the same pot, combine the carrots, zucchini, parsley, thyme, and pepper.

Cook, covered, over low heat for about 10 minutes, or until the veggies are tender.

Bring to a boil with the water.

Reduce the heat to medium-low and simmer for about 20 minutes, or until the veggies are soft. Remove the saucepan from the heat and allow it to cool slightly once you've finished cooking the veggies.

12 cup of the soup should be set away from the skillet.

Fill a blender halfway with soup and mix on low until smooth.

Cook, stirring constantly, until the pureed mixture and the held soup are hot.

Enjoy your meal!

Note: You may skip the blender stage if you like your veggies to remain whole.

Ingredients:

Soup made with chicken

4 quarts cubed chicken

6 oz.

1 hacked onion, half-cut

2 celery stalks, cut in half and slashed

1 cup carrots, peeled and cut in half

14 cup sliced parsley, cut in half 6 large garlic cloves, coarsely chopped

12 teaspoon black pepper (optional)

3 cup stock (chicken)

olive oil, 2 tablespoons

coconut flour, 2 tbsp

12 CUP CREAM OF COCONUT

seasonings to taste

In a small stockpot, combine the chicken, water, a large chunk of onion, celery, carrot, garlic, parsley, and dark pepper.

Toss the mixture in a pot with enough water to cover it and bring it to a boil.

Reduce the heat to low, cover, and cook for 45 minutes to an hour.

hour.

Through a colander, strain the stock into another saucepan.

5. Remove the cooked veggies from the pot and toss them out.

Set the pot aside after adding the chicken stock.

Heat the oil over medium heat in a large stockpot.

Mix in the flour, along with the remaining onion, celery, carrot, garlic, and parsley, for about 5-6 minutes, or until the onions are aromatic and clear.

Cook for about 1 minute, whisking constantly.

Now pour in the chicken stock, constantly stirring to avoid clumping.

Bring the mixture to a boil, then reduce to a low heat and simmer for another 8 minutes, or until delicate.

Cook until the cooked chicken and coconut milk are warmed through, then remove from the heat.

Season with salt and pepper to taste and serve at desired temperature.

Chapter Six

Paleo-Friendly Lobster Bisque

Lobster Bisque is a silky, creamy, and delectable soup. If you need another reason to make and eat this for lunch, make it a supper menu item. It's outstanding!

Ingredients:

4 tbsp. ghee/spread

2 tbsp. diced scallions

1 celery stalk, diced

coconut flour (four tablespoons)

PLUS: 2 CUP coconut milk, 2 teaspoons

tomato paste, 1 tablespoon

paprika, 2 tblsp.

1 tsp Old Bay

cayenne pepper (1/8 teaspoon)

2-3 tbsp. chicken stock

10 oz. deficient lobster meat, roughly chopped

to taste with salt and pepper

In a pan over medium low heat, melt the margarine.

Cook for 3 minutes, or until the scallions and celery have softened.

Toss the veggies with the coconut flour and combine well.

Cook for 3 minutes on medium heat, constantly mixing.

Pour the coconut milk slowly into the vegetable mixture and stir until well combined.

Combine the tomato paste and the other ingredients in a mixing bowl.

Cook for 5 minutes over medium-low heat, or until the bisque thickens.

Combine the paprika, Old Bay Seasoning, cayenne pepper, and broth in a large mixing bowl.

To combine the ingredients, mix them well.

Cooked lobster flesh should be added at this point.

To taste, season with salt and pepper.

Cook the bisque for an additional 5 minutes over low heat, or until it is thoroughly warmed.

Boiling is not recommended.

Now take a moment to savor each bite.

Tomato Basil Soup, Quick and Easy

3 huge tomatoes, peeled and diced

12 teaspoon oregano 1 onion, chopped

1/8 tsp marjoram

14 cup finely chopped new basil

2 cups stock made from chickens

to taste with salt and pepper

Directions:

In a medium-sized pot, combine the tomatoes, onions, garlic, oregano, marjoram, and basil. Bring to a boil with the chicken stock.

Reduce the heat to medium-low and cook for 20 minutes.

10 minutes of cooling

Pour the soup in small batches into a blender and puree until smooth.

For each batch, do the same.

Empty the soup into a new pot each time and reheat for a few moments before serving.

If desired, top with fresh basil.

Soup with chicken and vegetables that can be made quickly

1 cooked chicken, shredded after the meat has been removed.

12 red chili pepper, diced 12 red onion, finely chopped 4 enormous carrots, daintily sliced 12 enormous butternut squash, stripped and cubed

2 tblsp. garlic (minced)

1 tsp basil powder

1 tsp. oregano (dried)

lemon juice, 1 tablespoon

to taste with salt and pepper

Water that is fresh and cold

a few freshly hacked parsley branches

Directions:

In a large pot on the stove, combine the deconstructed chicken, celery, pepper, onion, carrots, squash, garlic, basil, oregano, lemon juice, salt, and pepper.

Make sure the chicken and vegetables are completely submerged in new virus water.

Cook, covered, on high for 20 to 30 minutes, or until the squash begins to mellow.

Stir in a handful of freshly slashed parsley before serving.

BEEF

a rub for roasting

You can't go wrong with a deliciously prepared piece of meat, and this one delivers.

Ingredients:

1 tsp. oregano (dried)

1 teaspoon garlic powder, 1 tablespoon sea salt

1 tsp chili powder

12 tsp. powdered onion

12 tsp cayenne pepper, powdered

paprika, 1 tblsp.

12 tsp. thyme (dried)

olive oil, 2 tablespoons

Broiler, 3–4 pound (toss and sirloin tip work well)

Preheat the oven to 350 degrees Fahrenheit and prepare the dish.

Use a stove-safe Dutch oven or line a baking sheet with aluminum foil.

In a small mixing bowl, combine oregano, salt, garlic powder, pepper, onion powder, cayenne, paprika, and thyme.

Stir in the olive oil until all of the ingredients are thoroughly combined.

Place the meat on a baking sheet that has been prepared ahead of time, and then brush the zest mixture on all sides of the meat.

Roast for 1 hour in a preheated oven, or until the dish reaches 145 degrees F on the inside.

Before slicing, let the meal rest for 15 to 20 minutes.

Meatloaf with a lot of meat in it

Paleostyle meatloaf is delectable in a variety of ways. You can also play with it. Try it in individual biscuit tins or a small bread portion dish. It looks like it'll be delicious in the end!

2 tbsp coconut oil (optional)

4 carrots, thinly sliced 1 onion (diced)

to taste with salt and pepper

1 to 2 teaspoons powdered bean stew

2 chopped chimine peppers

1 tblsp. Worcestershire sauce (made from scratch)

1 cup salsa (medium-hot)

3 lb. beef mince

beaten 3 eggs

Preheat the oven to 350°F and prepare the dish.

Heat the coconut oil over medium heat in a medium skillet.

Combine the carrots and onions in a large mixing bowl.

Salt, pepper, and bean stew powder are now added.

Cook, stirring occasionally, until the onion is translucent and the carrots begin to soften.

Sauté the ringer pepper until it begins to soften, about 2 minutes.

Cook for a couple of minutes longer with the Worcestershire sauce and salsa.

Allow to cool slightly after removing from heat.

Add the vegetable blend and eggs to the ground hamburger in a large mixing bowl.

Completely combine all ingredients.

Fill an 8" x 8" or 9" x 9" baking dish halfway with the ground meat mixture and shape into a loaf.

Bake for 1 hour or until the portion reaches 160 degrees F on the inside.

Remove the portion from the broiler and set aside for a few minutes before slicing.

Worcestershire Sauce (Made from Scratch):

Here's a Paleolithic topping you can make and keep on hand in case you come across a recipe that needs to be Paleolithic-ized.

1 cup vinegar from apple juice

coconut aminos (1/4 cup)

14 cup soy sauce (Thai) (discretionary, yet makes it taste great)

water (1/4 cup)

14 tsp. black pepper (coarse)

12 tsp. mustard (dried)

12 tsp. powdered onion

14 tsp. cinnamon powder

12 tsp ginger, powdered

12 tsp powdered garlic

In a pan on the stovetop, combine all of the ingredients.

Allow to simmer for 1 to 2 minutes after bringing to a boil.

Allow to cool before storing in a fridge compartment.

POULTRY

Buffalo Chicken that is made from scratch

Making your own chicken wings has the advantage of allowing you to make them as spicy or mild as you like.

Ingredients:

Wings or drumettes weighing 212 to 3 pounds

12 cup butter (ghee)

1 tsp. paprika (sweet)

1 tablespoon vinegar made from apple juice

2 finely minced garlic cloves

If you want a spicier sauce, add 4 tablespoons hot sauce or more.

Directions:

Preheat the broiler to 450°F or the grill to medium-high.

Clean the chicken pieces with a paper towel after rinsing.

In a small saucepan on the stovetop, melt the ghee over low heat.

In a large mixing bowl, combine the paprika, vinegar, garlic, and hot sauce.

Turn off the burner.

1/4 of the sauce should be poured into a small bowl, and the rest should be poured into a large mixing bowl and set aside.

Put the chicken pieces on a rimmed baking sheet lined with foil if you're using the broiler, or try a wire rack inside the rimmed baking sheet if you're using the oven. (The fat drips down through the rack and away from the chicken, resulting in crispier chicken.)

Brush the chicken with the sauce from the small bowl.

Cook the chicken pieces for 12-15 minutes on a medium-high heat setting if using a barbecue.

Prepare for 30 minutes under the broiler, turning halfway through.

After the chicken has finished cooking on the stove, turn on the broiler to sear and cook the wings on each side until they are crisp and dark.

Mix the cooked chicken pieces with the excess sauce in a large mixing bowl to coat them. Yummy!

Fajitas de Pollo de Pollo de Pollo De Pollo De Pollo

You won't miss the tortillas since these are so tasty. Actually, you may now focus on each of the recipe's fantastic tastes.

Ingredients:

chicken breasts weighing 2 pounds

1 tsp cumin 1 tsp bean stew mix

1 teaspoon pepper, freshly ground

To taste, season with salt

2 tbsp coconut oil

- cut chime peppers into strips (one of each shade)

makes for a delectable meal)

1 sweet onion, peeled and sliced into strips

1 medium jicama, peeled and sliced

3 mango pieces, peeled and peeled

3 quartered and peeled avocados

- 2 large lettuce leaves per head (margarine or Bibb lettuce works well)

1 bunch freshly cut cilantro

Instructions: Using a meat tenderizer, pound each chicken bosom piece until it reaches an equal thickness.

Cumin, stew powder, pepper, and salt should all be combined in a small basin.

In a container, heat 1-2 tablespoons coconut oil on medium.

Sprinkle a substantial amount of the flavors onto the pan once the oil is heated.

On top of the seasonings, place the chicken bosoms in the skillet.

On top of the chicken, sprinkle the remaining mixed flavors.

Sear the chicken's primary side for about 1 minute, then repeat with the other side.

Remove the chicken from the pan after it is cooked through and place it on a chopping board to cut into strips.

Cook the peppers and onions until they are soft on a similar griddle.

Turn off the heat after everything is done cooking.

Fill each dish with lettuce leaves.

Then, on top of the lettuce, arrange the sautéed peppers and onions, as well as the jicama, avocado, and mango slices.

On top, arrange the chicken parts.

PORK

Pork

Loaf

Instead of beef, pork is used in this delicious "meatloaf." I believe you will like the taste, and you may even come to prefer it over beef.

Ingredients:

1 lb. pork mince

beaten 1 egg

Almond flour, 4 teaspoons

coconut milk (1 cup)

a pinch of salt

12 tsp. cayenne

coconut oil (1 tablespoon)

1 finely chopped onion

6 entire, sliced mushrooms

Preheat the oven to 400 degrees Fahrenheit (200 degrees Celsius).

In a large mixing bowl, whisk together the ground pork, egg, almond flour, coconut milk, salt, and pepper.

Refrigerate for approximately 15 minutes after combining the ingredients.

Heat up the coconut oil in a frying pan over medium heat.

Add the onion and mushrooms to the heated oil and sauté until they are softened.

Remove the meat mixture from the fridge and stir in the sautéed onion and mushrooms.

Shape the dough into a loaf in an ungreased baking pan.

Bake for 1 hour in the oven. (Check for doneness in the middle.)

Allow a few minutes for cooling before slicing to desired thickness.

Pork Chops, Sweet and Salty

4 bone-in pork chops, seasoned to taste with salt & pepper

coconut oil, 4 teaspoons

sliced onions (two huge onions)

peeled, cored, and cut 4 apples

Directions:

Sprinkle salt and pepper on both sides of the pork chops.

2 tablespoons coconut oil in a large frying pan set over medium heat

Cook for 5 minutes on each side in the hot oil.

Remove the pork chops from the pan and put aside after they have browned.

Reduce the heat to medium-low in the frying pan and add the remaining 2 tablespoons of coconut oil.

The onions and apple slices should now be added.

Cook until the apple pieces are tender and the onions have caramelized.

Serve the pork chops with the apple-onion combination on the side.

SEAFOOD AND FISH Spaghetti with Shrimp

1 spaghetti squash Ingredients:

olive oil, 4 teaspoons

4 finely minced garlic cloves

1 tsp basil powder

shrimp (1 pound)

To taste, season with salt

Preheat the oven to 375 degrees Fahrenheit (190 degrees Celsius).

Cut the squash lengthwise in half using a long, sharp knife.

Remove the seeds using a scraping motion.

Apply a little olive oil to the squash's flesh.

Cook for 40-45 minutes with the squash facing down in a baking dish.

Pour the remaining olive oil into a frying skillet while the squash is cooking.

2 garlic cloves, minced, sauté till gently brown in olive oil over medium heat.

Remove the garlic and oil from the pan and set aside in a small bowl. (Toss this in with the squash after it's done.)

Allow the spaghetti squash to cool slightly once it has done cooking so that you don't get burnt while handling it.

Heat the remaining 2 tablespoons of olive oil in the frying pan while the squash is cooling.

Cook until the shrimp are done, then add the remaining 2 garlic cloves, basil, and shrimp.

When the frying pan is completed, turn off the heat beneath it.

Scrape the squash flesh into a large mixing basin using a fork. (It'll have a spaghetti-like consistency.)

In a large mixing bowl, combine the spaghetti with the remaining olive oil and garlic combination. 15. Arrange the shrimp on top of the "spaghetti" in serving plates.

Lemon-Salmon Salad

1 lemon's juice

2 tbsp walnut oil 1 tbsp lemon zest

4 salmon fillets, fresh or frozen 1 teaspoon dried dill 2 minced garlic cloves

salt from the ocean

Mix the lemon juice, lemon zest, walnut oil, dried dill, and garlic cloves together in a large mixing bowl.

Fill a gallon-sized Ziploc bag with the ingredients.

In a Ziploc bag, marinate the salmon fillets for 1 hour.

Preheat oven to 450 degrees Fahrenheit.

Remove the salmon fillets from the bag and lay them skin side down on an ungreased baking sheet.

Salt and pepper the fish fillets.

For 15-20 minutes, bake the salmon in the center of the oven.

Take the oven out of the equation.

Enjoy the salmon after removing the skin.

Gumbo with two kinds of meats

If you prefer gumbo foods with a kick, feel free to add some more spice to this recipe.

Ingredients:

olive oil, 2 tablespoons

8 oz. mushrooms, coarsely sliced 1 onion

4 tablespoons lime juice 1 pound boneless, skinless chicken, cubed

lemon juice, 3 teaspoons

basil (12 teaspoon)

12 teaspoon oregano (oregano, oregano, oregano, or thyme (12 teaspoon)

garlic, minced 1 tablespoon

1 tomato paste can (6 oz.)

14 cup tomatoes that have been sun dried

cooked shrimp (1 pound)

Instructions: Heat the olive oil in a large frying pan over medium heat.

In a large mixing bowl, combine the chopped onion, mushrooms, and chicken cubes.

Toss the spices and garlic into the pan with the lime and lemon juice.

Stir thoroughly, then cover and reduce to a low heat, stirring regularly, for about 12 to 15 minutes.

Add the tomato paste and dried tomatoes after the onions have softened and the chicken has cooked.

Stir until you have a sauce.

Reduce the heat to low and simmer, stirring periodically, for 10 to 15 minutes.

Stir in the shrimp and cook for a few minutes.

Serve the shrimp onto dishes after they're done cooking.

Fish seasoned with lemon pepper

This dish will appeal to anybody who dislikes the flavor of fish that has been cooked till it is dry. It adds moisture and taste to your fish.

two fillets of white fish

pepper (1 teaspoon)

1 lemon (12 oz. juice)

8 slices lemon

Seasonings in ghee or butter

Start by bringing some water to a boil in the bottom portion of the saucepan for this recipe, which is similar to how you would steam vegetables.

Cut two sheets of foil, each large enough to surround a fish fillet completely.

Each piece of foil should contain a fish fillet.

Season the fish with pepper, lemon juice, and four thin lemon slices on top of each piece.

Toss some small slices of butter on top of each fish to taste.

Wrap the foil around each piece of fish and secure the ends.

Cook for 20 minutes with the foil-wrapped fish pieces in the steamer top.

Each fish fillet should be carefully unwrapped and served with a vegetable or salad side dish.

Flounder with a Twist

Chapter Seven

Flounder with a Twist

I f you prefer "crunch" as much as I do, you'll love the nutty taste of this fish.

Ingredients:

4 eggs - 1 cup pecans, crushed in a food processor into a meal or whirlpool

6 fillets defrosted white fish

a pinch of salt

pepper (12 teaspoon)

14 teaspoon powdered garlic

12 cup pecans, chopped 2 teaspoons fresh parsley

Preheat the oven to 400 degrees Fahrenheit (200 degrees Celsius).

Whip the eggs in a basin large enough to dip the fillets into while the oven is preheating.

Combine the pecan meal, salt, and garlic powder in a bowl.

Using a big platter, pour the pecan mixture.

Coat each side of the fish with pecan meal after dipping it in the egg mixture.

In a large baking dish, carefully put each piece of fish.

Place any leftover pecan meal on top of the fish and pat it down once it has been placed in the dish.

Fresh parsley and chopped nuts should be added to the top.

Bake for 15-20 minutes after placing the baking dish in the oven. With a fork, check to see whether the fish is fully cooked and flaky.

Enjoy your meal!

Crab Cakes are a delicious treat.

Crab is one of my favorite foods, and these breadless crab cakes are the way to go. This dish allows you to savor the delicious flavor of crabmeat. You won't be able to eat crab cakes in any other manner after trying them.

1 pound fresh or canned crab meat

2 tbsp red onion, diced 2 tbsp chopped parsley

homemade 2 tbsp Mayonnaise made using paleo ingredients.

1 garlic clove, minced

to taste with salt and pepper

cayenne pepper (1/8 teaspoon)

1 ovary

coconut flour, 2 tbsp

3 to 4 tbsp. coconut oil

Fill a medium-sized mixing bowl halfway with crabmeat.

Combine the onion, parsley, mayonnaise, garlic, salt, pepper, cayenne pepper, egg, and flour in a mixing bowl.

To prevent the crab flesh from falling apart, stir thoroughly but gently.

Heat the coconut oil over medium heat in a large skillet.

Form patties out of the ingredients by dividing it into 10 equal amounts.

Allow the cakes to brown for about 2 to 3 minutes on each side.

Paleo Mayonnaise Instructions

Here's a Paleo mayo recipe you'll want to make again and again!

Ingredients:

2 tbsp. lemon juice, freshly squeezed

2 oz.

1 tablespoon mustard powder

To taste, salt 1 tsp.

cayenne pepper, 1/4 teaspoon (optional)

2 c. extra virgin olive

Directions:

Lemon juice, eggs, dry mustard, salt, and cayenne pepper should all be blended together in a blender (if using)

Pulse for a few seconds until foamy.

Allow your blender to run on low for a while.

Slowly drizzle in the oil until it emulsifies, practically a drop at a time.

Slowly drizzle in the oil until it's fully incorporated.

To taste, season with salt

Refrigerate the ingredients in a jar.

Ingredients:

Shrimp Salad with a Variety of Colors

cooked and peeled shrimp (1 pound)

3 to 4 ripe avocados, peeled and diced into 12 inch pieces

1 orange bell pepper, chopped 3-4 ripe tomatoes 2-3 green onions, neatly chopped 1 jalapeño pepper, seeded and coarsely chopped

3 to 4 minced garlic cloves

two limes' juice

Olive oil is a kind of vegetable oil that comes

finely sliced cilantro leaves

to taste with salt and pepper

Directions:

Combine the shrimp, avocados, tomatoes, onions, bell pepper, jalapeno pepper, and garlic in a large mixing bowl and gently combine.

Toss the salad with the lime juice and olive oil.

Season with salt and pepper to taste, then top with fresh cilantro.

Gently incorporate the ingredients.

Salmon with Nuts Baked

The combination of the softness of the salmon and the crunchiness of the coating creates a sensory treat to appreciate.

12 cup almond meal 1 pound skinless salmon fillet (almonds pulsed in a food processor)

12 cup chopped almonds

12 teaspoon powdered coriander 3 tablespoons fresh chives (chopped)

12 tsp cumin powder

1 lemon, juiced

to taste with salt and pepper

Coconut oil is a kind of vegetable oil that comes

cilantro, chopped (optional)

Preheat the oven to 350 degrees Fahrenheit (180 degrees Celsius).

Add the almond meal, almond pieces, chives, coriander, and cumin to a small mixing dish and stir to combine.

Season salmon fillets with salt and pepper after squeezing the lemon juice over them.

Using the almond meal mixture, coat both sides of each fillet.

Place the fillets skin side down on a lightly oiled broiler pan.

Bake for 12-15 minutes, checking with a fork to see whether the salmon flakes easily. If preferred, serve with fresh cilantro on top before serving.

APPETIZERS

Cukes with a Roll

Cucumber slices are quite simple to prepare using a mandolin slicer. Plus, you may add carrots and almonds to this filling if you like.

1 can tuna (12 oz)

lemon juice, 1 tbsp

handmade 14 cup Mayonnaise dating back to the Paleolithic period

dill weed (12 tbsp.)

to taste with salt and pepper

cucumbers, two big

Directions:

Mix the tuna, lemon juice, mayonnaise, dill weed, salt, and pepper together well in a small bowl.

Cucumbers should be washed and dried outdoors.

Place a cucumber lengthwise and slice using a mandolin slicer.

Place a little quantity of tuna mixture on one end of a cucumber slice and wrap it up like a sushi roll.

Carry on in this way until the tuna combination is completely depleted.

Ingredients:

Roll-ups de deli

Greek yogurt, plain (8 oz) (if you eat dairy)

12 cup cranberries (dried, unsweetened)

1 pound of cooked pork, sliced 12 cup pecans or walnuts, chopped

Fill a small mixing dish halfway with yogurt and set aside.

Toss in the nuts and dried cranberries.

Spread desired amount of filling on one end of a piece of meat flat on a plate.

Make a sushi roll out of it.

If desired, cut into small pieces.

Baby Bellas with a Stuffing

16 baby bella mushrooms are used as the main ingredient.

14 cup bell pepper, chopped 2–3 tablespoons olive oil

2 finely minced garlic cloves

1 lemon (zest) 1 onion (chopped)

a defrosted and drained 10 ounce box of frozen spinach

14 CUP NUTS (CRUMBLED) (almonds, pecans, walnuts)

1 cup shredded aged cheddar (optional)

14 cup olive oil and vinegar dressing, season to taste with salt and pepper

Directions:

Preheat your oven to 375 degrees Fahrenheit (190 degrees Celsius).

After that, chop up the mushroom stems.

1 tablespoon olive oil 1 tablespoon olive oil 1 tablespoon olive oil 1 tablespoon olive oil 1 tablespoon olive oil 1 tablespoon olive oil 1 tablespoon olive oil 1 tablespoon olive oil 1 tablespoon olive oil 1 tablespoon olive

Cook for 5 minutes with the bell pepper, onion, and garlic.

Reduce the heat to low and stir in the lemon zest, spinach, nuts, 12 cup cheese, salt, and pepper, along with the dressing.

Cook until the mixture has reached a satisfactory temperature.

Brush each mushroom cap with olive oil and place it in a baking dish with sides that has been lightly greased. 8. Fill each mushroom cap with a heaping spoonful of filling and top with the remaining cheese.

9. Bake for 20 minutes, or until the mushrooms are tender, in your preheated oven.

Cinnamon-Fruit Salad

peeled and diced 1 large orange

12 cup pecans or walnuts, chopped 1 teaspoon ground cinnamon 1 apple, diced 2 spears fresh pineapple, cubed 6–8 large strawberries, tops removed and sliced

12 CUP UNSWEETENED COCONUT SHREDGING (optional)

Directions:

In a medium bowl, combine the cut fruit.

Chopped nuts and cinnamon should be sprinkled on top.

Eggs with Avocado

Ingredients:

Hard-boiled eggs (four)

1 peeled, pitted, and diced avocado

2 tsp. chili powder

lemon juice (1 teaspoon)

to taste with salt and pepper

Directions:

Hard-boiled eggs should be peeled and cut lengthwise into halves.

Remove the yolks from the eggs and place them in a small bowl with the avocado cubes.

Smash the avocados and egg yolks together with a fork to make a paste.

In a large mixing bowl, combine the hot sauce, lemon juice, salt, and pepper.

Pour the yolk mixture back into the egg whites.

Sweet Potato Fries that have been baked

Ingredients:

14 cup oil (olive or coconut) 3 large sweet potatoes

2 teaspoons pumpkin pie spice, 1 tablespoon sea salt

2 tsp. Cajun spice

Directions:

Preheat the oven to 425 degrees Fahrenheit (200 degrees Celsius).

Sweet potatoes should be peeled and the ends cut off.

To make sticks, cut the potatoes in half lengthwise and cut them into rounded disks.

In a large mixing bowl, combine the sweet potatoes and oil.

To moisten the potatoes, combine all of the ingredients in a large mixing bowl and stir well.

Toss the salt, pumpkin pie spice, and Cajun seasoning together in a small mixing bowl.

Completely combine all ingredients.

In the same bowl as the potatoes, sprinkle the spices and mix well with your hands.

On a baking sheet, place a rack.

Make a single layer of sweet potatoes on the rack. There will be no need to turn the potatoes because the heat will circulate around them.

Bake until golden brown, about 25–30 minutes.

Allow for some cooling time before serving the potatoes.

Ingredients:

Shrimp Kabobs are a quick and easy dish to prepare.

a quarter cup of sesame oil

lemon juice (2 teaspoons)

garlic, minced 1 tablespoon

14 teaspoon ground black pepper

1 peeled pound of shrimp

Pour the oil, lemon juice, garlic, and pepper into a medium-sized mixing bowl.

Completely combine all ingredients.

In a large Ziploc bag, put the marinade.

Clean the shrimp by rinsing them and drying them with a towel.

Refrigerate the shrimp for at least two hours after putting them in the Ziploc bag.

Preheat the grill to a medium setting.

Put shrimp on individual skewers while the grill is heating up.

Place the skewers on the grill after it has heated up.

Cook the shrimp for 5 minutes, or until pink. (If the shrimp are overcooked, they will become tough.) Serve and enjoy!

Apple Crisp without the Bake

12 cup fresh-squeezed orange juice 4 apple slices, chopped

a third of a cup of chopped pecans

a third of a cup of walnuts, sliced

a third of a cup (34 cups) of golden raisins

1 t. ginger powder

1tsp cinnamon powder

nutmeg (1 tsp.)

Directions:

In an 8" x 8" baking dish, arrange the apples.

Over the apples, pour the orange juice.

Toss the apples in the mixture until they're completely covered.

Pulse the pecans, walnuts, raisins, ginger, cinnamon, and nutmeg until coarsely chopped in a food processor.

Serve with a dollop of nut mixture on top of the apple mixture.

Ingredients:

Cobbler (Blackberry)

1 pint blackberries (fresh or frozen)

14 c. honey (raw)

a quarter-cup of almond flour

arrowroot powder (12 teaspoon)

12 tbsp. baking soda 12 tbsp. salt

1 tbsp flour

1tsp cinnamon powder

1 tsp. nutmeg, freshly ground

12 cup coconut or almond milk

1 tsp vanilla

Preheat the oven to 350 degrees Fahrenheit (180 degrees Celsius).

Use olive or coconut oil to lightly grease an 8" x 8" baking dish.

Drizzle the honey over the blackberries in a baking dish.

Almond flour, arrowroot, salt, baking soda, baking powder, cinnamon, and nutmeg should all be combined in a separate bowl.

Combine the dry ingredients with the almond or coconut milk and vanilla extract.

If the batter is too dry, add more milk gradually until it reaches a smooth consistency.

Place the blackberries on top of the batter and bake it.

25–30 minutes in the oven

When the crust is browned, remove it from the oven. Enjoy!

Crust Ingredients for Banana Chocolate Pie:

a total of 12 cup almond flour

5 dates, chopped finely

1 tsp. salt

coconut oil (3 tablespoons)

Filling

5 bananas, peeled and sliced

5 chopped large dates

coconut milk (1 cup)

13 c. cacao powder, unsweetened

12 cup sliced almonds 1 tablespoon vanilla extract

2 oz. finely chopped dark chocolate

Directions:

Preheat the oven to 350 degrees Fahrenheit (180 degrees Celsius).

Using olive oil cooking spray or coconut oil, lightly coat a 9-inch pie pan.

A food processor is used to combine the almond flour, dates, and salt.

Pulse the dates and almond flour together until smooth.

Continue to process until the mixture forms a dough-like consistency. (If the mixture is too dry, add a few drops of oil until you achieve the desired consistency.)

Bake for 15 minutes, or until the crust is browned, pressing the dough into the pie pan.

While you make the filling, let it cool completely.

To make the filling, in a food processor, combine the bananas, dates, coconut milk, cacao powder, and vanilla.

Combine the ingredients in a blender and process until smooth.

Fill your cooled piecrust with the mixture and sprinkle the almonds and chocolate chips on top.

Cover with saran wrap and chill for at least 4 hours.

Remove the pie from the refrigerator about 30 minutes before serving, remove the cling wrap, and allow it to come to room temperature before slicing.

Enjoy your meal!

Donuts du chocolat

Ingredients:

Dates with pits (10)

2 tbsp vanilla extract 1 tbsp water

6 eggs are required.

12 CUP CONTAINED COCONUT FAT

12 tsp. cinnamon powder

14 tsp. salt from the sea

14 tsp. bicarbonate of soda

13 c. cacao powder, unsweetened

12 CUP COCONUT OIL, WHICH HAS BEEN REMOVED

Dark chocolate that's melted (72 percent or higher)

Directions:

Preheat the oven to 350 degrees Fahrenheit (180 degrees Celsius).

Using coconut oil, generously coat a doughnut skillet.

Microwave for 30 seconds on high in a microwave-safe bowl with the dates and water.

Remove the dates from the microwave and mash them into a paste with your hands.

Add the dates, glue, vanilla, and eggs to your food processor bowl.

Combine all ingredients in a blender and process until smooth.

In a separate bowl, combine the flour, cinnamon, salt, baking powder, cacao powder, and dissolved oil.

Mix and scrape down the sides of the processor as needed to achieve a smooth consistency.

Fill the dish circles to about 2/3 full with the mixture.

Place the player under the broiler for 15 to 20 minutes, or until it is fully cooked.

Remove the container from the heat and allow it to cool for 15 minutes on a cooling rack.

Remove the doughnuts from the skillet with care and set them to cool completely on a cooling rack.

If desired, garnish with liquefied chocolate or a favorite garnish.

Crust of C.C.C. Bars

12 pitted and de-seeded dried dates

14 cup crushed unsweetened coconut 12 cup almond butter

2 tsp honey (raw)

3 tbsp cacao powder (not sweetened)

1tsp cinnamon powder

sea salt, a pinch

Caramel

12 dried dates that have been hollowed out and soaked in water for an hour

6 tbsp. coconut milk (from a can)

water, 3 tbsp

1 tbsp vanilla essence (unadulterated)

sea salt, a pinch

Topping

1 cup softened dingy chocolate (72 percent or higher)

14 c. coconut milk (in a can)

2 tsp. coffee, ground

Toss with coarse salt and serve.

Directions:

Begin by sprinkling coconut or olive oil on a bread skillet.

Add all of the ingredients for your outside layer to a food processor: dates, almond butter, coconut, honey, cacao powder, cinnamon, and a pinch of salt.

Empty the mixture into your bread pan and solidly pack it into the lower part of the container with an even thickness throughout once it has completely consolidated.

Make the caramel as directed.

In a food processor, combine the dates and pulse until they separate. It takes about 45 seconds to complete this task.

While the processor is running, drizzle in the coconut milk little by little.

In the same manner, add the water.

Combine the vanilla extract and a pinch of salt in a small mixing bowl.

Handle the mixture until it resembles caramel. It should take between 4 and 5 minutes to complete the interaction.

Pour the caramel over the outside and spread evenly once you've achieved the perfect consistency.

Now, add the coconut milk to your dissolved chocolate.

To keep the chocolate pourable, microwave it for 30 seconds.

Blend in the espresso powder with the chocolate.

Pour the mixture over the caramel and spread it out with a tender touch to achieve an even layer.

On top of the chocolate, sprinkling some salt

To allow the chocolate to solidify, place your bread skillet in the refrigerator. After 15 minutes, this should occur. Enjoy the slices!

Coconut Pudding with Chocolate

Ingredients:

1 coconut milk (14 ounce) can

Almond milk (312 cup)

arrowroot powder (seven tblsp.)

9 tbsp. cacao powder (dark, unsweetened)

12 cup sugar made from coconut

2 tsp vanilla extract, pure and unadulterated

sea salt, a pinch

Topping of unsweetened shredded coconut

Directions:

Bring the coconut milk, almond milk, arrowroot powder, cacao powder, and sugar to a boil in a medium pot over medium-high heat.

Allow 2 minutes for the mixture to bubble, constantly blending. (The mixture should be thick in appearance.)

Add the vanilla extract and salt and mix well.

Fill dessert bowls halfway with the mixture.

Serve with shredded coconut on top as a garnish.

Bars with lemon

Ingredients: Topping

6 eggs are required.

8 lemons, 12 cup crude honey (1 cup)

12 CUP COCONUT OLIVE OLIVE OLIVE OLIVE O

Topping of unsweetened shredded coconut

Crust

1 cup almonds in their natural state

macadamia nuts (1 cup)

14 c. honey, unprocessed

2 eggs, melted 12 cup coconut oil

Directions:

Preheat the oven to 400 degrees Fahrenheit (200 degrees Celsius).

In a medium saucepan over medium-high heat, combine the eggs, honey, and lemon juice.

Toss in the coconut oil at this point.

Mix until the mixture thickens and bubbles.

Turn off the burner.

Place the mixture in a bowl in the refrigerator to cool. 7. Blend the almonds and macadamia nuts together in a food processor. 8. Pulse the nuts in short bursts until they're in small lumps. If you process the mixture too much, you'll end up with flour. The texture should be coarse and thick.

Place the nut mixture, honey, softened oil, and eggs in a blending bowl and blend until smooth.

Prepare a rectangular pan with coconut or olive oil. 11. Evenly distribute the mixture in the pan.

12. Bake for 15 to 20 minutes, or until the top layer is golden brown. 13. Turn off the heat and allow to cool completely.

Remove the lemon mixture from the cooler and spread it over the crust once the hull has cooled.

Return to the refrigerator if desired, with a sprinkling of shredded coconut on top.

Cut and eat when completely cool.

Refrigerate if not using right away.

Chapter Eight

Shrimp Kabobs

Shrimp Kabobs are a quick and easy dish to prepare.

a quarter cup of sesame oil

lemon juice (2 teaspoons)

garlic, minced 1 tablespoon

14 teaspoon ground black pepper

1 peeled pound of shrimp

Pour the oil, lemon juice, garlic, and pepper into a medium-sized mixing bowl.

Completely combine all ingredients.

In a large Ziploc bag, put the marinade.

Clean the shrimp by rinsing them and drying them with a towel.

Refrigerate the shrimp for at least two hours after putting them in the Ziploc bag.

Preheat the grill to a medium setting.

Put shrimp on individual skewers while the grill is heating up.

Place the skewers on the grill after it has heated up.

Cook the shrimp for 5 minutes, or until pink. (If the shrimp are overcooked, they will become tough.) Serve and enjoy!

Apple Crisp without the Bake

12 cup fresh-squeezed orange juice 4 apple slices, chopped

a third of a cup of chopped pecans

a third of a cup of walnuts, sliced

a third of a cup (34 cups) of golden raisins

1 t. ginger powder

1tsp cinnamon powder

nutmeg (1 tsp.)

Directions:

In an 8" x 8" baking dish, arrange the apples.

Over the apples, pour the orange juice.

Toss the apples in the mixture until they're completely covered.

Pulse the pecans, walnuts, raisins, ginger, cinnamon, and nutmeg until coarsely chopped in a food processor.

Serve with a dollop of nut mixture on top of the apple mixture.

Ingredients:

Cobbler (Blackberry)

1 pint blackberries (fresh or frozen)

14 c. honey (raw)

a quarter-cup of almond flour

arrowroot powder (12 teaspoon)

12 tbsp. baking soda 12 tbsp. salt

1 tbsp flour

1tsp cinnamon powder

1 tsp. nutmeg, freshly ground

12 cup coconut or almond milk

1 tsp vanilla

Preheat the oven to 350 degrees Fahrenheit (180 degrees Celsius).

Use olive or coconut oil to lightly grease an 8" x 8" baking dish.

Drizzle the honey over the blackberries in a baking dish.

Almond flour, arrowroot, salt, baking soda, baking powder, cinnamon, and nutmeg should all be combined in a separate bowl.

Combine the dry ingredients with the almond or coconut milk and vanilla extract.

If the batter is too dry, add more milk gradually until it reaches a smooth consistency.

Place the blackberries on top of the batter and bake it.

25–30 minutes in the oven

When the crust is browned, remove it from the oven. Enjoy!

Crust Ingredients for Banana Chocolate Pie:

a total of 12 cup almond flour

5 dates, chopped finely

1 tsp. salt

coconut oil (3 tablespoons)

Filling

5 bananas, peeled and sliced

5 chopped large dates

coconut milk (1 cup)

13 c. cacao powder, unsweetened

12 cup sliced almonds 1 tablespoon vanilla extract

2 oz. finely chopped dark chocolate

Directions:

Preheat the oven to 350 degrees Fahrenheit (180 degrees Celsius).

Using olive oil cooking spray or coconut oil, lightly coat a 9-inch pie pan.

A food processor is used to combine the almond flour, dates, and salt.

Pulse the dates and almond flour together until smooth.

Continue to process until the mixture forms a dough-like consistency. (If the mixture is too dry, add a few drops of oil until you achieve the desired consistency.)

Bake for 15 minutes, or until the crust is browned, pressing the dough into the pie pan.

While you make the filling, let it cool completely.

To make the filling, in a food processor, combine the bananas, dates, coconut milk, cacao powder, and vanilla.

Combine the ingredients in a blender and process until smooth.

Fill your cooled piecrust with the mixture and sprinkle the almonds and chocolate chips on top.

Cover with saran wrap and chill for at least 4 hours.

Remove the pie from the refrigerator about 30 minutes before serving, remove the cling wrap, and allow it to come to room temperature before slicing.

Enjoy your meal!

Donuts du chocolat

Ingredients:

Dates with pits (10)

2 tbsp vanilla extract 1 tbsp water

6 eggs are required.

12 CUP CONTAINED COCONUT FAT

12 tsp. cinnamon powder

14 tsp. salt from the sea

14 tsp. bicarbonate of soda

13 c. cacao powder, unsweetened

12 CUP COCONUT OIL, WHICH HAS BEEN REMOVED

Dark chocolate that's melted (72 percent or higher)

Directions:

Preheat the oven to 350 degrees Fahrenheit (180 degrees Celsius).

Using coconut oil, generously coat a doughnut skillet.

Microwave for 30 seconds on high in a microwave-safe bowl with the dates and water.

Remove the dates from the microwave and mash them into a paste with your hands.

Add the dates, glue, vanilla, and eggs to your food processor bowl.

Combine all ingredients in a blender and process until smooth.

In a separate bowl, combine the flour, cinnamon, salt, baking powder, cacao powder, and dissolved oil.

Mix and scrape down the sides of the processor as needed to achieve a smooth consistency.

Fill the dish circles to about 2/3 full with the mixture.

Place the player under the broiler for 15 to 20 minutes, or until it is fully cooked.

Remove the container from the heat and allow it to cool for 15 minutes on a cooling rack.

Remove the doughnuts from the skillet with care and set them to cool completely on a cooling rack.

If desired, garnish with liquefied chocolate or a favorite garnish.

Crust of C.C.C. Bars

12 pitted and de-seeded dried dates

14 cup crushed unsweetened coconut 12 cup almond butter

2 tsp honey (raw)

3 tbsp cacao powder (not sweetened)

1tsp cinnamon powder

sea salt, a pinch

Caramel

12 dried dates that have been hollowed out and soaked in water for an hour

6 tbsp. coconut milk (from a can)

water, 3 tbsp

1 tbsp vanilla essence (unadulterated)

sea salt, a pinch

Topping

1 cup softened dingy chocolate (72 percent or higher)

14 c. coconut milk (in a can)

2 tsp. coffee, ground

Toss with coarse salt and serve.

Directions:

Begin by sprinkling coconut or olive oil on a bread skillet.

Add all of the ingredients for your outside layer to a food processor: dates, almond butter, coconut, honey, cacao powder, cinnamon, and a pinch of salt.

Empty the mixture into your bread pan and solidly pack it into the lower part of the container with an even thickness throughout once it has completely consolidated.

Make the caramel as directed.

In a food processor, combine the dates and pulse until they separate. It takes about 45 seconds to complete this task.

While the processor is running, drizzle in the coconut milk little by little.

In the same manner, add the water.

Combine the vanilla extract and a pinch of salt in a small mixing bowl.

Handle the mixture until it resembles caramel. It should take between 4 and 5 minutes to complete the interaction.

Pour the caramel over the outside and spread evenly once you've achieved the perfect consistency.

Now, add the coconut milk to your dissolved chocolate.

To keep the chocolate pourable, microwave it for 30 seconds.

Blend in the espresso powder with the chocolate.

Pour the mixture over the caramel and spread it out with a tender touch to achieve an even layer.

On top of the chocolate, sprinkling some salt

To allow the chocolate to solidify, place your bread skillet in the refrigerator. After 15 minutes, this should occur. Enjoy the slices!

Coconut Pudding with Chocolate

Ingredients:

1 coconut milk (14 ounce) can

Almond milk (312 cup)

arrowroot powder (seven tblsp.)

9 tbsp. cacao powder (dark, unsweetened)

12 cup sugar made from coconut

2 tsp vanilla extract, pure and unadulterated

sea salt, a pinch

Topping of unsweetened shredded coconut

Directions:

Bring the coconut milk, almond milk, arrowroot powder, cacao powder, and sugar to a boil in a medium pot over medium-high heat.

Allow 2 minutes for the mixture to bubble, constantly blending. (The mixture should be thick in appearance.)

Add the vanilla extract and salt and mix well.

Fill dessert bowls halfway with the mixture.

Serve with shredded coconut on top as a garnish.

Bars with lemon

Ingredients: Topping

6 eggs are required.

8 lemons, 12 cup crude honey (1 cup)

12 CUP COCONUT OLIVE OLIVE OLIVE OLIVE O

Topping of unsweetened shredded coconut

Crust

1 cup almonds in their natural state

macadamia nuts (1 cup)

14 c. honey, unprocessed

2 eggs, melted 12 cup coconut oil

Directions:

Preheat the oven to 400 degrees Fahrenheit (200 degrees Celsius).

In a medium saucepan over medium-high heat, combine the eggs, honey, and lemon juice.

Toss in the coconut oil at this point.

Mix until the mixture thickens and bubbles.

Turn off the burner.

Place the mixture in a bowl in the refrigerator to cool. 7. Blend the almonds and macadamia nuts together in a food processor. 8. Pulse the nuts in short bursts until they're in small lumps. If you process the mixture too much, you'll end up with flour. The texture should be coarse and thick.

Place the nut mixture, honey, softened oil, and eggs in a blending bowl and blend until smooth.

Prepare a rectangular pan with coconut or olive oil. 11. Evenly distribute the mixture in the pan.

12. Bake for 15 to 20 minutes, or until the top layer is golden brown. 13. Turn off the heat and allow to cool completely.

Remove the lemon mixture from the cooler and spread it over the crust once the hull has cooled.

Return to the refrigerator if desired, with a sprinkling of shredded coconut on top.

Cut and eat when completely cool.

Refrigerate if not using right away.